Your Baby, Your Body, Your Journey

A Pregnancy hand book

By

Esther Bello

Table of content

Introduction

The Fluttering Begins

It starts with a flutter, a whisper in the deepest chambers of your being. A feeling, at first, so faint you could almost miss it. But it's there, a butterfly taking flight in the garden of your soul. You know, in that inexplicably certain way that women do, that something extraordinary has begun.

You're pregnant.

The word itself, "pregnant," carries the weight of a thousand suns. It's a universe contained within, a kaleidoscope of emotions, a symphony of changes, a dance of life unlike any other. It's a journey, yes, but it's also a metamorphosis. You are, quite literally, becoming something new.

This book is your compass on that journey. It's a map, meticulously crafted, to guide you through the twists and turns of pregnancy. It's a confidante, a friend who's been there, done that, and is here to tell you that you're not alone.

Within these pages, you'll find:

- The Science of Wonder: We'll delve into the fascinating biology of pregnancy, from the miracle of conception to the breathtaking development of your little one. You'll learn about the intricate dance of hormones, the cozy haven of your womb, and the awe-inspiring transformation of your body.

- The Symphony of Your Senses: Pregnancy is a sensory feast. We'll explore the rollercoaster of emotions, the sometimes-hilarious, sometimes-uncomfortable physical changes, and the newfound appreciation for the simple joys of life.

- The Choices That Matter: From prenatal care to birthing options, from nutrition to self-care, we'll empower you with the knowledge to make informed decisions about your pregnancy and your birth.

- The Strength Within: You are stronger than you know. This book will be your cheerleader, reminding you of your incredible resilience and the innate wisdom that resides within you.

But most importantly, this book is about you. It's about your baby, your body, and your unique journey. It's about celebrating the miracle of life, embracing the unknown, and trusting the incredible power that lies within you.

So, take a deep breath, mama-to-be. This is your story. Let's begin.

Chapter 1

The Seed Awakens - The First Trimester

The Fluttering: Announcement, Emotions, and Early Tweaks

It might start with a faint flutter, a whisper in your gut that sparks a knowing fire in your heart. Or, it could be a bold, blazing announcement: two pink lines staring back, confirming the secret your intuition already knew. Whatever your path, the news of pregnancy explodes into a kaleidoscope of emotions. Joy cartwheels with trepidation. Excitement tangles with uncertainty. It's a rollercoaster ride, and you're holding the ticket for the most thrilling adventure of your life.

This chapter welcomes you with open arms, holding space for every feeling that washes over you. We'll celebrate your announcement, whether it's a private whisper to your partner or a confetti-popping extravaganza with loved ones. We'll acknowledge the whirlwind of emotions, offering guidance on navigating anxieties and embracing the sheer wonder of it all. We'll talk about early physical changes, those little tweaks your body whispers about as it prepares for its incredible transformation.

Building a Home: Understanding Fetal Development and Maternal Changes

Welcome to the Womb: The First Four Weeks

- This stage is all about rapid cell division and laying the groundwork for your little one's future systems. From a single fertilized egg, a cluster of cells called a blastocyst forms, eventually implanting itself in the uterine lining.

- The neural tube, which will become the brain and spinal cord, begins to develop. This is a critical time, as any disruptions can lead to birth defects like spina bifida.

- Your body, meanwhile, gears up for this immense undertaking. Hormonal shifts cause morning sickness (or all-day sickness!), fatigue, and mood swings. But hey, these are signs your body is hard at work building a safe haven for your little one!

From Tadpole to Bean: Weeks Five to Eight

- This is where your little one starts looking distinctly human, albeit a very tiny human! The tadpole shape morphs into a recognizable baby with a head, trunk, and limb buds.

- The major organs, including the heart, lungs, kidneys, and digestive system, begin to form and function. Tiny fingers and toes sprout, though they might still be webbed, adding to the cuteness factor!

- You might start feeling flutters, the first movements of your baby! It's an electrifying moment, a sign that life is truly blossoming within you.

Growing Stronger: Weeks Nine to Twelve

- Your little bean is graduating to fetus now! All major organs are now present and functioning, laying the foundation for further growth and development.

- Bone formation accelerates, and the skeleton starts to solidify. Fingers and toes become distinct, losing their webbed appearance. Facial characteristics, such as eyes, nose, and mouth, take on greater clarity.

- You might be feeling more energetic now as the initial wave of morning sickness recedes. Embrace this newfound energy to stay active and take care of yourself!

Building a Double Dwelling: Understanding Twin Fetal Development and Maternal Changes in the First Trimester

First Trimester Twists: Doubling the Fun (and Maybe the Nausea!)

Carrying twins throws a few exciting curveballs into the first trimester experience. You might notice symptoms kicking in earlier and feeling more intense. Morning sickness? Try double the nausea, double the fatigue, double the cravings (and maybe the aversions!). But hey, with double the joy coming your way, it's all part of the remarkable journey.

The Double Domino Effect: Witnessing Twin Development

Imagine two tiny universes blossoming within you, developing side-by-side in your cozy womb. This section dives into the fascinating details of twin development during the first trimester. We'll explore two possible scenarios:

- Monozygotic Twins: These twins arise from a single fertilized egg splitting in two, resulting in identical babies with the same sex and shared genetic material. We'll follow their incredible journey from a single blastocyst to two distinct bean-shaped fetuses with their own amniotic sacs and placentas.

- Dizygotic Twins: These twins result from the fertilization of two separate eggs, making them fraternal twins with potentially different sexes and unique genetic profiles. We'll witness the magic of two separate fertilized eggs implanting in the uterine wall, each embarking on its own individual, yet parallel, developmental journey.

More to Feel, More to Bond With: Unique Experiences in a Twin Pregnancy

Carrying twins in the first trimester can bring heightened emotional experiences. You might feel overwhelmed at times, but the joy and excitement are often doubled too. We'll discuss:

- Early Movement Sensations: Some women carrying twins report feeling movement earlier than singleton pregnancies. Imagine the thrill of feeling two fluttering sparks instead of one!

- Increased Fundal Height: Your uterus might grow faster, leading to earlier bump visibility. Embrace the double dose of adorableness!

- Enhanced Maternal Intuition: With two little lives entrusted to you, your nurturing instincts might kick in even stronger.

Navigating the Double Dose: Adapting Prenatal Care and Lifestyle

Twin pregnancy often requires more frequent prenatal checkups and additional monitoring. We'll talk about:

- Early Scans and Tests: You might have additional ultrasounds or blood tests to confirm twin pregnancy and monitor their development.

- Dietary Adjustments: Your nutritional needs double, so ensuring proper intake of essential nutrients becomes crucial.

- Exercise Modifications: Staying active is important, but you might need to adjust your exercise routine to accommodate your growing twins.

Building a Support System for Your Double Journey

Carrying twins can be both physically and emotionally demanding. This section emphasizes the importance of building a strong support system:

- Connecting with other Twin Moms: Sharing experiences and advice with other mothers of twins can be invaluable. We'll provide resources for finding online communities and in-person support groups.
- Communicating with Your Partner and Family: Open communication and shared responsibility are key.

Fueling for Double: Embracing Your Nutritional Needs

Think of your diet as the building blocks for your baby's development. This is where we break down the essential nutrients you need and tips for incorporating them into your meals:

- Folate: This superhero nutrient helps prevent birth defects like spina bifida. Load up on leafy greens, fortified cereals, and lentils.
- Iron: Your blood volume increases in pregnancy, and iron carries oxygen to both you and your baby. Lean meats, fish, beans, and iron-fortified foods are your friends.
- Calcium: For strong bones and teeth, calcium is your best buddy. Dairy

products, dark leafy greens, and calcium-fortified foods are the way to go.

- Protein: Essential for building tissues and muscles, protein should be a regular guest on your plate. Choose lean meat, eggs, dairy, nuts, and legumes.

- Healthy Fats: Don't shy away from good fats! They keep you satiated, fuel your baby's brain development, and contribute to nutrient absorption. Opt for avocado, nuts, seeds, and incorporate olive oil into your choices.

Remember, listen to your body! Cravings? Indulge in moderation. Feeling nauseous? Stick to smaller, bland meals and don't hesitate to talk to your doctor about managing morning sickness.

Moving in Rhythm: Safe and Effective Exercises for the First Trimester

Engaging in physical activity benefits not only you but also your baby! It boosts your mood, energy levels, and sleep quality, while promoting healthy blood flow and preventing pregnancy discomforts. Here are some gentle and effective exercises to embrace:

- Walking: Lace up your shoes and get those endorphins flowing! Walks in nature are especially rejuvenating.
- Prenatal Yoga: Stretching and breathing exercises in a supportive

environment can work wonders for your body and mind.

- Swimming: The buoyancy of water is a blessing for your growing belly. Aqua aerobics classes can be a fun and refreshing option.
- Strength Training: Light dumbbell or bodyweight exercises help maintain muscle tone and prepare your body for postpartum recovery.

Pay attention to your body's cues and avoid exerting excessive pressure on yourself.

Always consult your doctor before starting any new exercise routine, especially if you have any health concerns.

The Art of Self-Care: Prioritizing Your Well-being

Pregnancy is a marathon, not a sprint, and self-care is your secret weapon. Here are some ways to replenish your energy and nurture your spirit:

- Prioritize Sleep: Your body needs extra rest to build a tiny human. Aim for 7-8 hours of sleep each night, and don't hesitate to take naps if you need them.
- Connect with Nature: Immerse yourself in the calming beauty of nature. Take a stroll in the park, tune into the birdsong, or just inhale the crisp, fresh air.
- Embrace Relaxation Techniques: Meditation, deep breathing exercises, and prenatal massages can help manage stress and anxiety.

- Spend Time with Loved Ones: Surround yourself with positive people who support you and uplift your spirits. Sharing your journey with them can be incredibly comforting.
- Pamper Yourself: Take a long bath, read a good book, or indulge in a spa treatment. You deserve it!

Remember, self-care isn't selfish, it's essential. By taking care of yourself, you're taking care of your baby too. Don't be afraid to ask for help and delegate tasks when you need to. This is your time to bloom, mama, and self-care is the sunshine that nourishes your beautiful journey.

Navigating the Uncharted: Prenatal Care, Tests, and Addressing Concerns in the First Trimester

The first trimester throws a whirlwind of new experiences your way, and navigating the medical unknowns can feel overwhelming. Worry not, mama-to-be! This chapter is your compass, guiding you through the labyrinth of prenatal care, tests, and potential concerns like a seasoned adventurer.

Unveiling the Map: Establishing Prenatal Care

Prenatal care is your lifeline throughout pregnancy, ensuring your health and your little one's well-being. Here's what to expect:

- Finding the Right Doctor: Choose a provider you feel comfortable with, someone who listens to your concerns and respects your decisions. Ask trusted friends for recommendations, read online reviews, and schedule introductory appointments to find the perfect fit.
- Early Checkups: Expect frequent visits in the first trimester, establishing baselines for your health and monitoring your baby's development. These visits include physical exams, blood tests, and early ultrasounds.
- Open Communication: Don't shy away from asking questions or

voicing concerns. Your doctor is there to support you, so speak up about anything that worries you, however big or small.

Demystifying the Maze: Understanding Common First-Trimester Tests

Tests in the first trimester paint a picture of you and your baby's health. Here are some common ones:

- Nuchal Translucency Scan: This ultrasound looks for markers of chromosomal abnormalities like Down syndrome.
- Combined First-Trimester Screening: This combines blood tests and an

ultrasound to assess the risk of chromosomal abnormalities.

- Non-invasive Prenatal Testing (NIPT): This advanced blood test screens for chromosomal abnormalities with high accuracy.

Remember, each test has its benefits and limitations. Discuss your options with your doctor to make informed decisions based on your personal preferences and risk factors.

Conquering the Unforeseen: Addressing Concerns and Managing Anxieties

The first trimester is a rollercoaster of emotions, and worries are bound to pop up. Here's how to tackle them:

- Morning Sickness: Don't let the name fool you, it can last all day! Ginger, bland foods, and small, frequent meals can offer relief. Talk to your doctor about medication if needed.

- Fatigue: Listen to your body and nap when you can. Prioritize sleep and delegate tasks to avoid burnout.

- Anxiety and Stress: Talk to your doctor or therapist about healthy coping mechanisms like exercise, meditation, or deep breathing exercises.

- Spotting and Cramping: Some spotting is normal, especially early on. However, any significant bleeding or severe pain warrants immediate medical attention.

Remember, you're not alone in this journey. Lean on your doctor, partner, family, and friends for support. Don't hesitate to reach out for help, whether it's for managing physical discomfort or navigating emotional challenges.

Conquering Discomforts:

- Morning Sickness: This all-day nemesis can knock you for a loop. Try ginger (tea, candy, even raw!), small, frequent meals, bland foods, and staying hydrated. Don't forget, acupressure wristbands and even ice chips can be your secret weapons.

- Fatigue: Listen to your body! Prioritize rest, delegate tasks, and embrace naps. Gentle exercise like walking or prenatal yoga can boost energy too. Remember, fatigue is temporary, and those extra Zzz's are building a tiny masterpiece!

- Mood Swings: Hormones are on a rollercoaster, and emotions may follow suit. Talk to loved ones, find healthy outlets like journaling or creative pursuits, and don't be afraid to seek professional help if needed. Remember, it's okay to not feel okay sometimes.

- Aching Body: Pregnancy comes with its own set of aches and pains. Warm baths, light stretches, and prenatal massages can offer relief. Consider a supportive maternity belt for back pain, and consult your doctor for any persistent discomfort.

Tackling Fatigue:

- Fuel Your Body: Eating a balanced diet rich in whole grains, protein, and fruits/vegetables gives your body the energy it craves. Stay hydrated to keep your internal engine running smoothly.

- Give importance to rest: Strive for 7-8 hours of restful sleep every night.Establish a relaxing bedtime routine, invest in blackout curtains, and avoid screens before bed. Remember, naps are your friends!

- Move Your Body: Gentle exercise like walking, swimming, or prenatal yoga can boost energy levels and improve mood. Find activities you enjoy and listen to your body's signals.

- Delegate and Ask for Help: Don't be afraid to ask family and friends for assistance with chores, errands, or childcare. This is a time to lean on your support system and allow yourself to rest.

Finding Joy in the Transformation:

- Celebrate the Little Things: Notice the first flutters, the growing bump, and the newfound connection with your little one. Each milestone is a reason to celebrate, even the seemingly small ones.
- Reconnect with Nature: Go for walks in the park, listen to the birdsong, and soak up the sunshine. Being in

nature can be incredibly grounding and uplifting.

- Nourish Your Creativity: Express yourself through writing, painting, music, or any creative outlet that brings you joy. Pregnancy is a time for personal growth and exploration.

- Connect with Other Moms: Share your experiences and find support in online communities or local parent groups. Knowing you're not alone can make a world of difference.

- Focus on Gratitude: Practice gratitude for your body, your baby, and the incredible journey you're on. Keeping a gratitude journal can enhance your well-being and remind you of the blessings surrounding you.

Remember, the first trimester is just the beginning of your incredible adventure. It's a time of change, challenges, and yes, even joy. By embracing the discomforts, managing your energy, and finding moments of delight, you can navigate this exciting phase with grace and confidence.

Chapter 2:

Blossoming Strength - The Second Trimester

Finding Your Rhythm: Embracing the Energy Surge and Body Confidence

Energy Surge:

- The second trimester often brings a welcome resurgence of energy after the initial fatigue of the first trimester. This is due to hormonal fluctuations and stabilization of the placenta.

- Embrace this energy by engaging in activities you enjoy, whether it's exercise, creative pursuits, or spending time with loved ones. Tune in to your body's signals and adapt your activities accordingly.

- Prioritize a balanced diet and adequate sleep to fuel your energy and ensure well-being.

Body Confidence:

- The second trimester marks a period of rapid fetal growth, often accompanied by a noticeable bump. This physical change can trigger a range of emotions, including joy, excitement, and sometimes insecurity.
- Practice self-compassion and positive body image affirmations. Focus on the incredible transformation your body is undergoing and the miracle of life it's creating.
- Surround yourself with supportive individuals who celebrate your

pregnancy and appreciate your body in all its stages. Consider joining a pregnancy support group or prenatal yoga class to connect with other expectant mothers.

Remember:

- Every woman experiences pregnancy differently. The timing and intensity of energy surges and body confidence shifts can vary.
- There is no "one size fits all" approach to navigating these changes. Be patient with yourself and prioritize your physical and emotional well-being.
- Do not hesitate to seek support from your healthcare provider if you have any concerns or questions about your

physical or mental health during pregnancy.

Baby on the Move: Feeling Kicks, Understanding Growth, and Bonding with Your Bump

Those were flutters in the first trimester, but now? Welcome to the kickboxing party! Tiny limbs pummel your insides, sending waves of joy and amusement. Each kick is a conversation, a secret code only you and your little one understand. Talk to your bump, sing, play music, and feel the connection deepen with every playful jab.

Growth continues in leaps and bounds (literally!). Learn about the amazing developments happening inside you: tiny fingers and toes flexing, lungs practicing their first breaths, and a brain forming intricate pathways. This knowledge sparks awe, fosters a deeper bond, and makes you marvel at the silent symphony playing within.

Choices and Decisions: Birthing Options, Prenatal Classes, and Planning for Arrival

Ah, the moment of decision arrives! This exciting chapter equips you with the knowledge and guidance needed to navigate the world of choices that come with birthing and welcoming your little one. Buckle up, mama, because it's time to personalize your journey!

Birthing Options: Charting Your Course:

- Hospital Birth: The traditional setting, offering extensive medical resources and pain management options. Consider if immediate medical intervention is desired, access to specialists is crucial, or if the comfort of a dedicated medical team is paramount.

- Birth Center: A home-like environment specializing in natural births with limited medical intervention. Explore if you prefer a more intimate setting, prioritize minimal interventions, and have a low-risk pregnancy.

- Home Birth: Bringing your baby Earthside in the comfort of your own space. Requires careful planning, a supportive team of midwives and doulas, and a low-risk pregnancy with open communication with your healthcare provider.

Prenatal Classes: Empowering Your Knowledge:

- Childbirth Education: Learn about stages of labor, pain management techniques, breathing exercises, and fetal development. Explore various birthing positions and comfort measures to equip yourself for the big day.
- Breastfeeding Support: Get expert guidance on latching, positioning, and troubleshooting challenges for a smooth breastfeeding journey.
- Newborn Care: Acquire the practical skills of diapering, bathing, feeding,

and soothing your little one with confidence.

- Sibling Preparation: Help your older children adjust to the arrival of their new sibling through fun activities and open communication.

Planning for Arrival: Nesting with a Nudge:

- Creating a Nursery: Carve out a cozy haven for your newborn, considering comfort, functionality, and your personal style. Invest in essentials like a crib, changing table, and feeding supplies.
- Packing Your Hospital Bag: Pack for yourself and your baby, including comfortable clothes, toiletries, nursing essentials, and

entertainment for longer stays. Don't forget diapers, wipes, and baby outfits!

- Stocking Up: Prepare for postpartum life with groceries, diapers, wipes, breastfeeding supplies, and medications to avoid last-minute scrambling.
- Financial Considerations: Discuss budgeting for childcare, maternity leave, and potential medical expenses with your partner. Delve into insurance possibilities and discover financial aid alternatives.

Remember:

- There's no "right" choice for any of these decisions. Your birthing experience, prenatal education, and arrival preparations should be tailored to your unique needs and preferences.

- Open communication with your healthcare provider is key. Discuss your options, ask questions, and voice your concerns to make informed decisions you feel confident about.

- Embrace the adventure! This is a once-in-a-lifetime journey, filled with exciting choices and countless possibilities. Trust your instincts, enjoy the process, and welcome your little one with open arms!

Building Your Nest: Preparing for Baby, Nesting Instincts, and Home Transformations

Nesting Instincts: A Primal Urge to Prepare:

As the second trimester unfolds, a surge of nesting instincts may kick in. This primal urge, shared across animal and human kingdoms, is all about creating a safe and comfortable environment for your baby. Don't resist it, embrace it!

Preparing for Baby: From Practicalities to Pampering:

- Nursery Creation: This is your chance to unleash your inner designer! Whether you prefer a minimalist modern vibe or a whimsical wonderland, create a space that reflects your personality and nurtures your baby's senses. Invest in essentials like a crib, changing table, rocking chair, and storage solutions.

- Gathering Gear: Stock up on practical essentials like diapers, wipes, baby clothes, feeding supplies, and bath products. Don't forget the fun stuff - books, toys, and cuddly blankets to create a stimulating environment.

- Pamper Yourself: Nesting isn't just about the baby! Take time to pamper yourself amidst the preparations.

Indulge in prenatal massages, relaxing baths, or simply curling up with a good book. Remember, a happy mama makes a happy baby!

Home Transformations: Big or Small, Changes Welcome Your Baby:

- Safety First: Ensure your home is baby-proofed by securing electrical outlets, removing tripping hazards, and installing gates. Consider child-proofing cabinets and drawers to keep curious hands safe.

- Comfort and Functionality: Think about how you'll move and interact with your baby in different spaces. Create a designated feeding area with comfortable seating and easy access to supplies. Optimize your bathroom for diaper changes with a changing table and storage for essentials.

- Embrace Your Style: Don't feel pressured to transform your entire home into a nursery. Incorporate baby-friendly touches while maintaining your own space and personality. Hang beautiful artwork, add cozy throws and pillows, and personalize your space to reflect your family's unique vibe.

Remember:

- Nesting is a natural and personal experience.Trust your instincts and follow what resonates best with you.
- Don't be afraid to ask for help! Delegate tasks, involve your partner

and family, and seek support from
friends or professionals if needed.

- Most importantly, enjoy the process!
Creating a welcoming haven for your
baby is a beautiful way to express
your love and anticipation.

Chapter 3:

The Transformation - The Third Trimester

The Home Stretch: Facing Fatigue, Discomfort, and Anticipation

Facing Fatigue: Embracing Rest and Prioritizing Sleep:

- The third trimester often brings a return of fatigue, as your growing baby demands more energy. Listen to your body, mama! Prioritize rest, delegate tasks, and embrace naps whenever possible.

- Invest in comfy clothes and supportive pillows to ensure comfortable sleep at night. Remember, a well-rested mama is a happy and healthy mama.

Discomfort and Adjustments: Navigating Body Changes and Aches:

- Backaches, leg cramps, and swelling are common companions in the third trimester. Talk to your healthcare provider about safe strategies for managing discomfort, such as prenatal massages, stretches, and supportive garments.

- Embrace body positivity! Your changing body is incredible, creating and nurturing a tiny miracle. Focus on the amazing feats your body is accomplishing, and treat yourself with kindness and compassion.

Anticipation and Excitement: Preparing for Your Baby's Arrival:

- This is the time to finalize birthing plans, pack your hospital bag, and ensure everything is prepped for your little one's arrival. Channel your nesting instincts to organize the nursery, wash baby clothes, and stock up on essentials.
- Connect with your baby through gentle belly rubs, soothing music,

and positive affirmations. Talk, sing, and read aloud, creating a loving bond even before your first meeting.

Remember:

- Every woman experiences the third trimester differently. Some sail through, while others face more challenges. Take your time and focus on taking care of yourself.
- Communication is key! Don't hesitate to discuss any concerns or discomforts with your healthcare provider. They're by your side, offering support throughout your journey.
- Embrace the excitement! This is a magical time of anticipation and preparation. Savor the moments,

celebrate your journey, and welcome your little one with open arms.

Preparing for Takeoff: Learning Birth Signaling, Pain Management, and Delivery Options

The third trimester is a time of intense anticipation, sprinkled with a healthy dose of nesting instincts and, of course, preparation for the big event: birth! This chapter equips you with the knowledge and tools to navigate the final leg of your pregnancy journey, focusing on birth signaling, pain management, and delivery options.

Birth Signaling: When is it Time to Launch?

Your body is an amazing communicator, sending out subtle (and sometimes not so subtle) signals that it's time to welcome your little one. Stay vigilant for these crucial signals:

- Regular contractions: These are rhythmic tightening and relaxing of the uterine muscles, becoming stronger and closer together as labor progresses.
- Bloody show: A pinkish or bloody mucus discharge indicating the loss of the mucus plug that sealed the cervix.

- Breaking of waters: A gush or trickle of clear or slightly pinkish fluid as the amniotic sac ruptures.

Breaking of waters during pregnancy

- Increased urge to nest: A sudden burst of energy to clean, organize, and prepare for the baby's arrival.
- Changes in baby movement: Less frequent or more intense movements can indicate the baby is settling into position for birth.

Pain Management: Choosing Your Comfort Zone

Labor pain is a natural part of the birthing process, but that doesn't mean you have to go it alone. Explore various pain management options to find what suits you best:

- Natural methods: Breathing exercises, relaxation techniques, massage, and warm compresses can help manage discomfort without medication.

Breathing exercises during pregnancy

- Medications: Epidurals, spinal blocks, and pain-relieving medications offer varying degrees of pain relief, with different risks and benefits to consider. Engage in a conversation with your healthcare professional to ensure an informed choice.

Delivery Options: Charting Your Course

The birthing experience is unique to each woman, and your delivery options should reflect your preferences and comfort level. Here are some common choices:

- Vaginal birth: The most traditional route, where the baby exits through the vagina. This can happen in a hospital, birth center, or even at home, depending on your healthcare provider and risk factors.

- Cesarean section (C-section): A surgical procedure where the baby is delivered through an incision in the abdomen. This may be necessary for medical reasons or if a vaginal birth is deemed unsafe.

- Cesarean section (Csection)
- Water birth: Delivering the baby in a pool of warm water, offering potential pain relief and a more natural birthing environment.

Remember:

- There is no "right" way to give birth. The most important thing is to choose a method that feels safe and comfortable for you and your baby.
- Talk openly and honestly with your healthcare provider about your preferences and concerns. They can guide you through the decision-making process and ensure

you have all the information you need.

- Trust your instincts and embrace the journey. Birth is a powerful and transformative experience, and you are strong and capable of birthing your baby in whatever way feels right for you.

The Empowered Birth: Understanding Your Choices, Building a Birth Team, and Trusting Your Intuition

Understanding Your Birth Choices:

- Informed Consent: You have the right to be informed about all your birthing options, including birthing locations, pain management methods, interventions, and potential complications. Ask questions, research thoroughly, and feel empowered to make decisions that align with your values and preferences.

- Birth Plans: Use these as flexible roadmaps, outlining your desires for labor and delivery. Include details like pain management preferences, birthing environment preferences, and newborn care practices. Remember, plans can adapt to circumstances, but serve as valuable communication tools with your healthcare team.

- Advocate for Yourself: Don't hesitate to voice your concerns or preferences throughout the birthing process. Ask questions, clarify information, and politely decline interventions you're not comfortable with.

Building a Birth Team:

- Healthcare Provider: Choose a provider who listens to your concerns, respects your choices, and supports your birthing vision. Explore options like OB-GYNs, midwives, or doulas depending on your needs and preferences.
- Doula: These non-medical birth companions offer emotional and physical support during labor and delivery. They can provide massage, breathing techniques, and advocacy, empowering you to have a positive birthing experience.

- Partner or Support Person: Choose someone who is calm, reliable, and supportive of your birthing choices. Their presence can offer comfort, encouragement, and practical assistance during labor.

Trusting Your Intuition:

- Listen to Your Body: Pay attention to your body's cues during labor. Rest when needed, move when you feel the urge, and trust your instincts about birthing positions and pain management.

- Embrace Your Emotions: Labor can be an emotional rollercoaster. Allow yourself to feel whatever arises, express your needs, and trust that your emotions are natural and valid.

- Believe in Yourself: You are strong and capable of birthing your baby. Trust your inner strength, focus on your breath, and visualize a positive birthing experience.

Remember:

- There is no "perfect" birth experience. Every woman and every birth is unique. Focus on creating a safe and supported environment where you can feel empowered and in control.
- Communication is key throughout the birthing process. Stay open with your healthcare team and support person, express your needs and concerns, and work together to create a positive and memorable experience.

- Celebrate your birthing journey, no matter how it unfolds. You are a warrior!

Welcoming Life: The Moment of Arrival, Postpartum Changes, and Embracing Motherhood

Welcoming Life" marks the culmination of your pregnancy journey with the momentous arrival of your little one. It also delves into the whirlwind of postpartum changes and the beautiful embrace of motherhood. Let's explore these exciting themes:

The Moment of Arrival:

- A Breathtaking Encounter: The first meeting with your baby is an experience etched in eternity. Witnessing their tiny features, feeling their delicate skin, and hearing their precious cries fills your heart with an overwhelming surge of love and wonder.

- Navigating the Delivery: Whether it's a smooth vaginal birth, a C-section, or anything in between, the moment of arrival is unique to each journey. Stay calm, focus on your breathing, and trust your healthcare team to guide you through the process.

- Instant Connection: The bond between mother and child blossoms instantly. From skin-to-skin contact to the first latch, each moment fosters a powerful connection that deepens with every passing day.

Postpartum Changes:

- Physical Transformations: Your body will undergo significant changes as it recovers from pregnancy and childbirth. Embrace these changes with self-compassion and celebrate your body's incredible feat of nurturing a life.
- Emotional Rollercoaster: Be prepared for a spectrum of emotions, from overwhelming joy to moments of vulnerability and fatigue. These ebbs and flows are normal, and seeking support from your partner, family, and healthcare provider is crucial.
- Newborn Needs: From feeding and sleep schedules to diaper changes

and soothing cries, life revolves around your newborn's needs. Embrace the learning curve, take things one step at a time, and don't hesitate to ask for help when needed.

Embracing Motherhood:

- Discovering New Strength: Motherhood unlocks a reservoir of strength you never knew you had. From late-night feedings to endless cuddles, each challenge fosters resilience and an unmatched ability to care for another being.
- Finding Joy in the Ordinary: Everyday moments become extraordinary with your little one. From bath time giggles to first smiles, cherish the simple joys and

discover the magic in every interaction.

- Building a Village: Lean on your support system – your partner, family, friends, and healthcare providers. You don't have to do this alone, and asking for help allows you to thrive in your new role as a mother.

Remember:

- Every mother's journey is unique. Don't compare yourself to others, embrace your own pace, and focus on building a strong foundation for yourself and your baby.
- Be gentle with yourself, both physically and emotionally. The postpartum period is a time for healing, rest, and adaptation. Listen

to your body and prioritize your well-being.

- Celebrate your motherhood! You are a miracle maker, a nurturer, and a fierce protector. Embrace the challenges, cherish the joys, and trust your instincts as you navigate this incredible new chapter in your life.

Chapter 4:

The Rhythm of Two - The First Weeks and Months

The Golden Hour: Skin-to-Skin Contact, Bonding with Your Newborn, and Breastfeeding Basics

Skin-to-Skin Contact:

- A Primal Connection: The first hour after birth, known as the "golden hour," is a sacred time for immediate skin-to-skin contact between mother and baby. This simple act fosters an incredible sense of connection, warmth, and security, regulating your baby's temperature, heart rate, and breathing.

- Hormonal Symphony: Skin-to-skin contact triggers a cascade of hormones in both mother and baby, promoting bonding and breastfeeding success. Oxytocin, the "love hormone," surges, fostering maternal instincts and calming anxieties.
- Nurturing the Bond: Beyond physiological benefits, skin-to-skin contact offers a powerful opportunity to bond with your baby. Listen to their heartbeat, smell their sweet

scent, and gaze into their eyes, establishing a connection that transcends words.

Bonding with Your Newborn:

- Getting to Know Each Other: The first weeks and months are a time of discovery and getting acquainted with your little one. Observe their unique quirks, listen to their cries, and respond to their needs with love and patience.

- Building a Secure Attachment: Every interaction, from feeding to diaper changes to simply singing a lullaby, contributes to building a secure attachment with your baby. This strong foundation lays the groundwork for emotional well-being and healthy development in the years to come.

- Embracing the Messy Magic: Motherhood is not always picture-perfect. Embrace the sleepless nights, the spit-up, and the unexpected tears. These messy moments are woven into the fabric of your unique bond, creating a lifetime of cherished memories.

Breastfeeding Basics:

- A Natural Partnership: Breastfeeding is a beautiful way to nourish your baby and strengthen your bond. However, it can also be challenging at first. Seek support from lactation consultants, join breastfeeding groups, and remember, every journey is unique.

- Learning Together: Don't be discouraged by initial difficulties. Latching, positioning, and milk supply can take time and practice. Be patient with yourself and your baby, and trust that you can learn to breastfeed together.

- Nourishment Beyond Milk: Breastfeeding offers much more than just nutrition. It provides antibodies that boost your baby's immune system, promotes healthy development, and creates a unique closeness that words cannot describe.

Remember:

- Every mother and baby's journey is unique. Some may bond instantly, while others take time. Embrace your own pace, prioritize skin-to-skin contact, and trust that your love will guide the way.

- Don't hesitate to seek support. From lactation consultants to experienced mothers, there are many resources available to help you navigate the challenges and joys of breastfeeding.

- Cherish these precious early days. The first weeks and months with your newborn are fleeting moments of pure wonder. Savor every interaction, capture the memories, and embrace the magic of this transformative chapter.

Finding Your New Normal: Factual Note on Sleep, Feeding, and Adjusting to Parenthood

Sleep Schedules:

- Newborn Sleep Patterns: Newborns have erratic sleep patterns, waking frequently to feed and be comforted. It's essential to adjust your expectations and prioritize rest whenever possible.

- Developing Routines: Gradually establish a bedtime routine with calming activities to signal sleep time. However, it's important to remember that consistent routines may take several months to become effective.

- Sharing Sleep Responsibilities: If you have a partner, share night-time duties to ensure both parents get adequate sleep. Consider safe co-sleeping practices, if desired, or invest in a bassinet near your bed for easy access.

Feeding Routines:

- Breastfeeding or Formula: Choose the feeding method that best suits your needs and preferences. Both breastfeeding and formula provide complete nutrition for your baby.
- Demand Feeding: Initially, feed your baby on demand, responding to their hunger cues rather than a strict

schedule. This helps establish good milk supply and promotes bonding.

- Gradual Routines: As your baby grows, you can introduce a more predictable feeding schedule with consistent intervals between meals. Consult your healthcare provider for guidance on specific feeding quantities and timings.

Adjusting to Parenthood:

- Embrace Change: Accept that your life will be different, and adapt to the ever-changing needs of your baby. Be patient with yourself and your little one as you navigate new routines and challenges.
- Seek Support: Don't hesitate to reach out for help from your partner, family, friends, or healthcare

professionals. Sharing your experiences and asking for support can alleviate stress and make you feel less alone.

- Focus on Self-Care: Prioritize your physical and emotional well-being. Eat healthy meals, get enough sleep, and engage in activities you enjoy.Keep in mind that a content and well-balanced parent is more adept at providing care for their child.

Remember:

- Every parent and baby's journey is unique. There's no "right" way to do things. Trust your instincts, seek support when needed, and allow yourself time to adjust to this transformative experience.

- Celebrate the small victories and cherish the precious moments with your little one. Parenthood is a rewarding journey filled with challenges and immense joy.

Emotional Rollercoaster: Diving into Baby Blues, Postpartum Support, and Building Community

Parenthood unfolds as a beautiful expedition, yet it doesn't consistently bask in rays of sunshine and rainbows. The first few months can be a whirlwind of emotions, and sometimes, the highs are met with unexpected lows. Let's explore the emotional rollercoaster of this time, focusing on recognizing baby blues, accessing postpartum support, and building a community of understanding.

Recognizing Baby Blues:

- Baby blues are a common experience affecting up to 80% of new mothers. They typically occur within the first few days to weeks after birth and can manifest in various ways:
    - Mood swings: Feeling sad, anxious, irritable, or tearful.
    - Difficulty sleeping or changes in appetite.
    - Overwhelming feelings of fatigue and exhaustion.
    - Difficulty bonding with your baby.
- Remember: Baby blues are different from postpartum depression (PPD). They usually resolve within a few

days or weeks with adequate rest, support, and self-care.

Seeking Postpartum Support:

- Reach out for help: If you're experiencing baby blues or suspect PPD, don't hesitate to seek support. Talk to your healthcare provider, a trusted friend or family member, or a mental health professional.
- Therapy or support groups: Consider individual therapy or joining support groups for new mothers to connect with others who understand your experiences and offer emotional support.

Building Community:

- Connect with other mothers: Surround yourself with positive and supportive people who can offer practical help and emotional validation. This could be joining a local new moms group, online communities, or even connecting with friends who are already mothers.

- Share your experiences: Talking openly about your emotions can be cathartic and help you feel less alone. Don't be afraid to share your challenges with trusted friends, family, or a therapist.

- Accept help and support: Don't be afraid to ask for help with daily tasks, childcare, or errands. This allows you time to focus on your well-being and bonding with your baby.

Remember:

- You are not alone. Many mothers experience emotional challenges after childbirth. It's important to reach out for help and build a supportive community around you.
- Prioritize self-care. Take time for activities you enjoy, get enough sleep, and eat healthy meals. Ensuring your well-being empowers you to provide optimal care for your little one.
- Celebrate the small victories. Motherhood is a journey filled with ups and downs. Be kind to yourself, celebrate even the smallest achievements, and trust that you are doing a great job.

Celebrating Milestones: Early Development, First Smiles, and the Joy of Every Moment

Welcome to the beautiful and rewarding journey of parenthood! Witnessing your baby's development unfold is a unique privilege, filled with countless milestones to celebrate, big and small. This note explores the importance of celebrating these achievements, focusing on early development, the magic of first smiles, and finding joy in every moment.

Early Development Milestones:

- Every baby develops at their own pace, but there are general milestones to look for in the first year:

- First few months: Head control, rolling over, reaching for objects, recognizing familiar faces.

- Six to nine months: Sitting unassisted, babbling, exploring with hands and mouth, showing emotions.

- Nine to twelve months: Crawling, pulling to stand, saying first words, understanding simple instructions.

- Celebrate each achievement: Every milestone, from the first head wobble to the first tentative steps, is a testament to your baby's incredible growth and learning. Acknowledge and celebrate these moments with joy and enthusiasm, fostering your baby's sense of accomplishment and confidence.

- Focus on the journey, not just the destination: Remember, development is a continuous process, not a race. Be present in each moment, enjoy the wonder of discovery in your baby's eyes, and celebrate the small victories along the way.

The Magic of the First Smile:

- There's nothing quite like the first smile from your baby. It's a magical moment of connection and pure joy, lighting up your heart and solidifying the bond between you.

- First smiles typically appear around six to eight weeks, though it can vary. When it happens, savor the moment! Capture it in a photo, share it with loved ones, and let it wash over you with happiness.

- Beyond the initial sparkle, smiles become a powerful tool for communication and emotional expression. Encourage your baby's smiles by mimicking their facial expressions, singing songs, and engaging in playful interactions.

Finding Joy in Every Moment:

- Parenthood is an experience filled with countless precious moments, often hidden in the ordinary: a giggle during bath time, a snuggle on the couch, the soft cooing of contentment.

- Train your eyes to see beauty everyday. Embrace the messy moments, the unexpected surprises, and the quiet joys of simply being present with your little one.
- Don't get caught up in the pressure to document every milestone on social media. Savor the moments privately, connect with your baby authentically, and create memories that will stay with you for a lifetime.

Remember:

- Celebrating milestones is not about comparing your baby to others. Embrace your child's unique journey and find joy in their individual pace and accomplishments.

- Most importantly, celebrate yourself! Becoming a parent is a transformative experience, filled with challenges and triumphs. Be kind to yourself, acknowledge your own growth, and celebrate the incredible role you play in your baby's life.

Chapter 5:

Forever Changed - Embracing Your New Identity

The Evolving Me: Redefining Self-Care, Rediscovering Passions, and Balancing Motherhood

The Evolving Me:

- Accepting the Change: Embrace the fact that you are no longer the same person you were before. You've evolved, acquired wisdom, and emerged resilient. This transformed version of yourself radiates beauty and capability

- Redefining Priorities: Motherhood brings a natural shift in priorities. Your needs and desires may take a backseat for a while, but that doesn't mean they disappear. Find ways to integrate your needs into your new life, even in small ways.

- Celebrating the Journey: Acknowledge the challenges and celebrate the victories. Becoming a new version of yourself is a journey, not a destination. Be patient, kind to yourself, and appreciate the progress you make every day.

Redefining Self-Care:

- Self-care is not a luxury, it's a necessity. It's not about bubble baths and massages (although those can be lovely!), it's about making choices that nourish your mind, body, and spirit.

- Find your new self-care rituals: What activities make you feel energized and fulfilled? Maybe it's a walk in nature, a phone call with a friend, or simply spending time reading a book. Prioritize these activities, even if it's just for a few minutes each day.

- Don't be afraid to ask for help: You can't pour from an empty cup. Allow your partner, family, and friends to support you so you can take some time for yourself and recharge.

Rediscovering Passions:

- Motherhood can often feel all-consuming, but it's important to hold onto your passions. What brought you joy before your baby arrived? Is it writing, painting, playing music, or pursuing a hobby?

- Find pockets of time: Even if it's just for a few minutes each day, make time for the things that make your soul sing. These activities can be your anchor, reminding you of who you are outside of motherhood.

- Embrace the unexpected: You may discover new passions during motherhood. Maybe you find joy in cooking healthy meals for your family, creating art with your child, or volunteering in your community.

Be open to new experiences and let your passions evolve alongside you.

Balancing Motherhood:

- Balance is a myth: Don't strive for a perfect balance because it doesn't exist. There will be days when motherhood takes over, and that's okay. The key is to be present and give your best to each moment, knowing that things will ebb and flow.

- Communicate and collaborate: Talk to your partner, family, and friends about your needs and expectations. Share responsibilities and delegate tasks so you can all share the load and support each other.

- Embrace the imperfections: There will be messy moments, missed deadlines, and days when you feel like you're failing. That's normal! Don't be afraid to laugh at yourself, learn from your mistakes, and focus on progress, not perfection.

Remember:

- Motherhood is a beautiful and challenging journey that will change you forever. Embrace the changes, redefine your priorities, and find ways to nurture your own needs alongside those of your child.
- There is no one right way to be a mother. Be true to yourself, listen to your instincts, and trust that you are doing the best you can.

- You are not alone. There are countless resources available to support you on this journey. Don't hesitate to reach out for help when you need it.

Growing Together: Nurturing Your Relationship, Communication, and Expanding Family

Nurturing Your Relationship:

- Shifting Roles and Responsibilities: Pregnancy and parenthood often bring changes to roles and responsibilities within a relationship.

Open communication and willingness to adapt are crucial to supporting each other and strengthening your bond.

- Maintaining Intimacy and Connection: While physical intimacy may take a backseat during pregnancy, finding new ways to connect emotionally and maintain intimacy is essential. This could involve shared activities, meaningful conversations, and simply expressing love and appreciation.

- Supporting Each Other: Parenthood brings its own set of challenges. Be there for each other, offer emotional and practical support, and remember that you're a team navigating this journey together.

Communication and Understanding:

- Open and Honest Communication: Clear and honest communication is vital throughout pregnancy and parenthood. Discuss your feelings, needs, and expectations openly, and make sure you both feel heard and understood.

- Managing Disagreements: Disagreements are inevitable, especially when sleep-deprived and navigating new terrain. Learn to communicate effectively, listen to each other's perspectives, and find solutions that work for both of you.

- Seeking Support Together: If you're struggling with communication or navigating challenges within your relationship, don't hesitate to seek professional help from a therapist or counselor specializing in couples and family issues.

Expanding Family:

- Welcoming a New Member: Adjusting to the arrival of a new baby can be challenging for both parents and existing family members. Allow time for everyone to adjust to the new dynamic and offer support to each other.

- Maintaining Individual Identities: While becoming parents is a significant change, remember to maintain your individual identities and interests outside of parenthood. This can help maintain a healthy balance and strengthen your individual well-being.

- Building Family Traditions: Creating new traditions and rituals can help foster a sense of family identity and belonging. This could involve anything from weekly family meals to celebrating special occasions together.

Remember:

- Every couple and family experiences pregnancy and parenthood differently. Be patient with yourselves and each other, embrace the changes, and focus on nurturing your relationship and supporting each other through this transformative journey.

Looking Ahead: Future Plans, Career Adjustments, and Embracing the Unfolding Journey

Looking Ahead: Navigating New Horizons

Career Adjustments:

- Redefining your career aspirations: Motherhood can spark a reevaluation of your professional goals. Consider flexible work options, exploring new fields, or even taking a career break to focus on family.

- Communication and negotiation: Discuss career plans with your partner and employer openly. Explore options like part-time schedules, remote work, or childcare solutions to bridge the gap between your professional ambitions and family needs.

- Investing in growth: Don't let parenthood halt your professional development. Seek upskilling opportunities, attend online courses, or build your network to keep your career path vibrant.

Crafting Future Plans:

- Dream beyond the immediate: While cherishing the present, allow yourself to envision the future you and your family desire. Picture your careers, interests, and goals intertwined with the joy of parenthood.

- Openness to possibilities: Embrace the fluidity of life. Unexpected turns and opportunities may arise, and being adaptable will allow you to navigate them with grace and enthusiasm.

- Flexibility and compromise: Building a future plan often involves compromise and adjustments. Discuss priorities with your partner and family, ensuring everyone feels heard and included in the crafting of your shared future.

Embracing the Unfolding Journey:

- Letting go of control: It's impossible to predict the future perfectly. Accept that unforeseen challenges and joys will be a part of your journey. Embrace the unknown with a spirit of adventure and trust your ability to adapt and thrive.

- Living in the present: Cherish the moments, both big and small, that define your motherhood experience. Savor the laughter, the cuddles, and the everyday magic of nurturing your little one.

- Finding fulfillment in the journey: While planning is important, remember that happiness often lies in the present moment. Find joy in the everyday aspects of motherhood, and trust that your journey will unfold beautifully, one precious moment at a time.

Remember:

- There's no single right way to navigate motherhood and career aspirations. Create a path that feels authentic and fulfilling for you, drawing strength from your support system and adapting as needed.
- Embrace the challenges and celebrate the victories, big and small. Motherhood is a journey of constant learning, growth, and unwavering love. Enjoy the present, plan for the future, and trust your intuition to guide you on this incredible adventure.

Reflections and Gratitude: Celebrating Your Strength, Cherishing Memories, and Embracing Unconditional Love

As your incredible journey nears its peak, it's time to pause and reflect on the extraordinary transformation you've undergone. This chapter is dedicated to celebrating your inner strength, cherishing the precious memories you've made, and opening your heart to the unparalleled love that awaits you.

Celebrate Your Strength:

- Acknowledge the physical, emotional, and mental resilience you've displayed throughout your pregnancy. Recall moments where you defied limitations, conquered fears, and embraced new challenges. Honor your body's remarkable ability to create and nurture life.

Cherish Your Memories:

- Take a moment to revisit the cherished moments that have etched themselves onto your soul. Remember the first flutter of movement, the awe-inspiring ultrasound images, and the outpouring of love and support from loved ones. Let these memories fill you with gratitude and anticipation.

Embrace Unconditional Love:

- Imagine the moment you first gaze into your newborn's eyes. Prepare your heart for the surge of overwhelming love, a love that knows no bounds and transcends all understanding. This unique, unconditional love will guide you and shape your journey as a mother.

Prompts for Self-Reflection:

- Consider writing a letter to your pregnant self, offering words of encouragement and celebrating your triumphs.

- Create a memory capsule for your future child, filled with mementos and messages that capture the essence of this extraordinary time.

- As you prepare to meet your little one, write down your hopes and dreams for your future together. Let these aspirations be your guiding light.

Remember:

- You are a warrior mama, strong, capable, and worthy of boundless love. Embrace this new chapter with open arms, knowing that you are never alone on this incredible journey.

This chapter is a springboard for reflection, gratitude, and self-discovery. Let it be a space to celebrate your remarkable strength, cherish the memories that have shaped you, and prepare your heart for the transformative power of unconditional love.

Conclusion: Your Triumphant Arrival

Dearest mama,

You've reached the final page of this guide, but know that the journey you've embarked upon has just begun. You've navigated months of transformation, embraced challenges with a warrior spirit, and nurtured a miracle within your very being.

You stand now on the precipice of parenthood, ready to meet your greatest adventure face-to-face.

Remember the early days, the flutter of awakening life, the thrill of witnessing your body's wondrous dance of creation? Hold onto those memories, the nervous excitement, the bursts of laughter, the quiet moments of awe. They are the threads woven into the tapestry of your journey, stories you'll share with your little one when they're ready to hear them.

This book was a companion, a map through uncharted territory. But the real guide has always been your intuition, your inner strength, the fierce love that has bloomed within you. Lean on these as you step into the world of parenthood. Trust your instincts, embrace the chaos, and celebrate every milestone, big or small.

Motherhood is an ever-evolving landscape, a path paved with both sunshine and tears. But through it all, remember: you are not alone. The village of love you built throughout your pregnancy remains by your side, a chorus of cheers and whispered wisdom. Lean on their shoulders, share your joys and fears, and find solace in their unwavering support.

As you cradle your newborn in your arms, a feeling unlike any other will wash over you. It's the culmination of every hope, every dream, every sleepless night. It's the fierce, boundless love that knows no limits, the love that whispers, "You are enough."

This love, mama, is your compass. It will guide you through late-night feedings, diaper explosions, and moments of doubt. It will fuel your patience, ignite your laughter, and become the foundation upon which you build your family.

So breathe deep, dear mama. You've walked through fire, danced with hormones, and birthed a miracle. Strength and capability define you, surrounded by an abundance of love. Go forth, embrace the wonder that awaits, and remember - the adventure has just begun.

With love and pride,l

Your guide and companion,

"Your Baby, Your Body, Your Journey"